MENOPAUSE DIET RECIPES FOR BEGINNERS

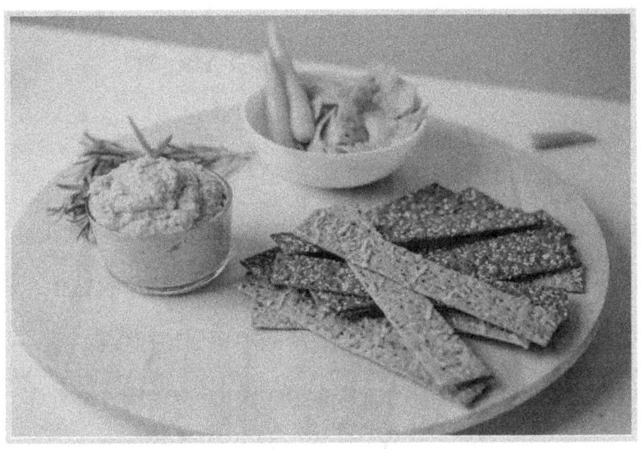

Healthy Eating For A

Symptom-Free Transition

Karla Mayer

Table Of Content

Introduction

Welcome to "Menopause Diet Recipes for Beginners," where we'll set out on a quest to empower women getting around the significant life transition of menopause. This phase, marked by hormonal fluctuations and various physiological changes, can often feel like uncharted territory. However, armed with the right knowledge and tools, this transition can be managed with grace and vitality.

Menopause is a natural biological process that every woman experiences as she reaches her late 40s or early 50s. It signifies the end of menstruation and fertility, accompanied by a multitude of symptoms ranging from hot flashes and night sweats to mood swings and weight gain. While these symptoms are a normal part of the menopausal journey, they can significantly impact a woman's quality of life.

One powerful tool in managing these symptoms is through a well-balanced diet tailored to the needs of menopausal women. This book is designed specifically for beginners, providing a comprehensive guide to understanding the role of diet in alleviating menopausal symptoms and promoting overall health and well-being.

In the following chapters, we will delve into the science behind menopause, exploring the physiological changes that occur and how they impact dietary needs. We will discuss the essential nutrients that menopausal women require to support hormonal balance and mitigate symptoms. From there, we will guide you through the process of creating a personalized menopause diet plan that fits your lifestyle and preferences.

Throughout the book, you will find a diverse array of recipes carefully crafted to nourish your body and soul during this transformative phase. From hearty breakfasts to satisfying dinners, energizing snacks to refreshing beverages, each recipe is designed with both taste and nutrition in mind.

Additionally, we will provide practical tips and strategies for meal planning and preparation, making it easier than ever to incorporate healthy eating habits into your daily routine. Whether you're cooking for yourself or feeding a family, our recipes are simple, delicious, and designed to support your journey through menopause.

As you embark on this culinary adventure, remember that you are not alone. With the right knowledge, tools, and support, you can embrace menopause with confidence and vitality. So let's dive in and discover the transformative power of food in managing menopause symptoms and embracing this new chapter of life with joy and resilience.

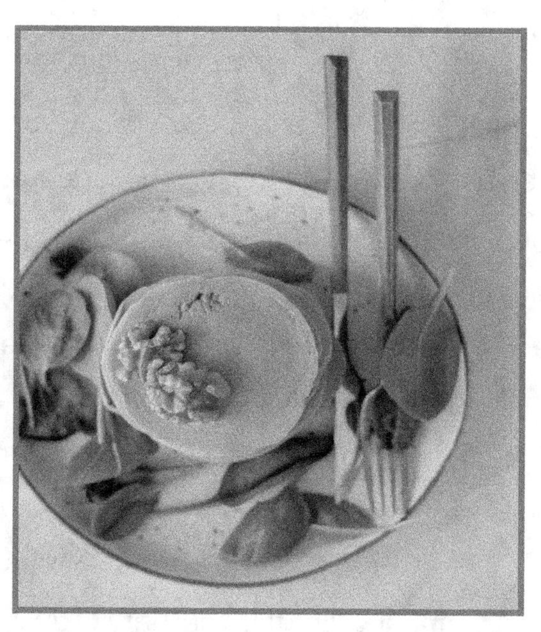

Chapter One

Understanding Menopause

In this chapter, we will delve into the fundamentals of menopause, exploring its definition, stages, and the physiological changes that occur within the body. Understanding menopause is crucial for women embarking on this transformative journey, as it provides the foundation for navigating through its challenges with grace and knowledge.

What is Menopause?

The end of a woman's reproductive years is marked by the normal biological process of menopause. It is defined as the cessation of menstruation for 12 consecutive months, signaling the end of ovulation and fertility. While menopause is often associated with women in their late 40s or early 50s, the age at which it occurs can vary widely among individuals. Some women may experience menopause earlier due to factors such as genetics, lifestyle, or medical interventions, while others may undergo it later in life.

Stages of Menopause:
Menopause is not a sudden event but rather a gradual transition marked by several stages:

Perimenopause: This phase typically begins several years before menopause, usually in a woman's 40s, but can start earlier for some. During perimenopause, hormonal fluctuations become more pronounced, leading to irregular menstrual cycles, changes in menstrual flow, and the onset of menopausal symptoms such as hot flashes, night sweats, mood swings, and fatigue. While fertility declines during perimenopause, pregnancy is still possible, so contraception may still be necessary for women not wishing to conceive.

Menopause: The stage of menopause is officially reached when a woman has gone 12 consecutive months without menstruating. At this point, ovarian function has ceased, and estrogen and progesterone levels decline significantly. Menopausal symptoms may continue during this stage, but they often lessen in severity over time.

Postmenopause: Postmenopause refers to the period following menopause. During this stage, menopausal symptoms may persist but usually diminish in intensity. However, women are still at risk for certain health issues associated with menopause, such as osteoporosis, heart disease, and cognitive decline, due to the prolonged decrease in estrogen levels.

Physiological Changes During Menopause:
Hormonal changes, specifically a decrease in the ovaries' production of progesterone and estrogen, are the main causes of menopause. These hormones play crucial roles in regulating the menstrual cycle, supporting reproductive function, and maintaining overall health.

As estrogen levels decline, women may experience a range of physical and emotional symptoms, including:

1. Hot flashes: Sudden feelings of intense heat, often accompanied by sweating and flushing of the face and neck.
2. Night sweats: Episodes of sweating during sleep, which can disrupt sleep patterns and contribute to fatigue.
3. Vaginal dryness: Reduced moisture and elasticity in the vaginal tissues, leading to discomfort during intercourse and an increased risk of urinary tract infections.
4. Mood swings: Fluctuations in mood, including irritability, anxiety, and depression, which can impact overall well-being and quality of life.
5. Changes in libido: Decreased interest in sexual activity due to hormonal fluctuations and physical discomfort.

In addition to these symptoms, menopause is also associated with changes in metabolism, body composition, and bone density, which can increase the risk of weight gain, muscle loss, and osteoporosis.

Understanding menopause is the first step toward going through this transformative journey with confidence and resilience. In the chapters that follow, we will delve deeper into the role of diet in managing menopausal symptoms and promoting overall health and well-being.

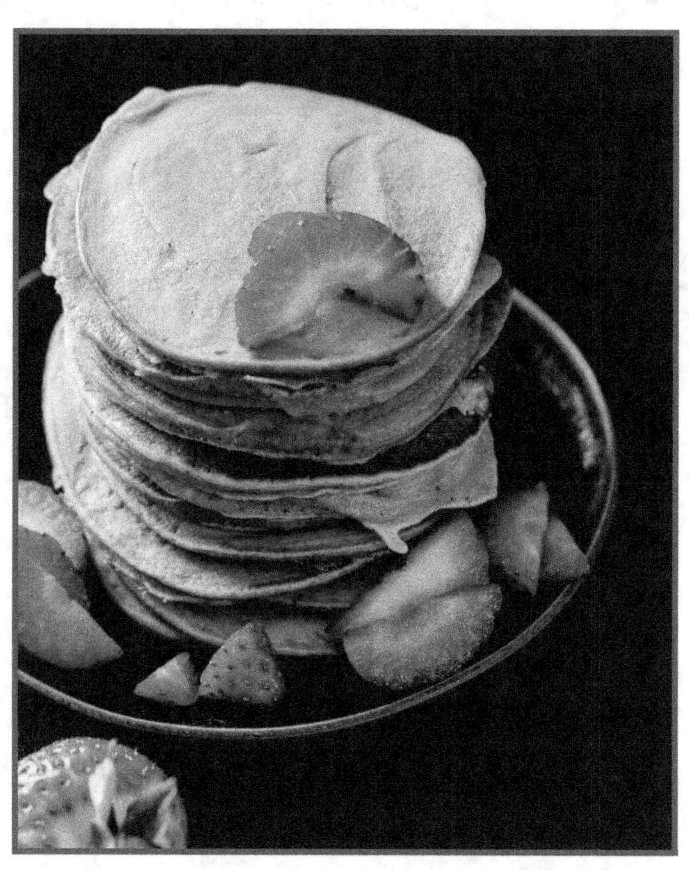

Chapter Two

The Role of Diet in Managing Menopause Symptoms

Here, we will explore the profound impact that diet can have on managing the symptoms associated with menopause. From hot flashes to mood swings, the foods we eat play a crucial role in alleviating discomfort and promoting overall well-being during this transitional phase of life.

Understanding Nutritional Needs During Menopause:

As women approach menopause, their nutritional needs undergo significant changes. Hormonal fluctuations, metabolic shifts, and changes in body composition all influence the body's requirements for essential nutrients. To effectively manage menopausal symptoms and support overall health, it is essential to focus on a diet that is rich in key nutrients while minimizing processed foods, sugar, and unhealthy fats.

Key Nutrients for Menopausal Women

Calcium and Vitamin D: Maintaining bone health becomes increasingly important during menopause, as estrogen levels decline, leading to a loss of bone density. Adequate intake of calcium and vitamin D is crucial for preserving bone strength and reducing the risk of osteoporosis and fractures. Good dietary sources of calcium include dairy products, leafy green vegetables, tofu, and fortified foods, while vitamin D can be obtained from sunlight exposure and supplementation.

Omega-3 Fatty Acids: Omega-3 fatty acids have anti-inflammatory properties and may help alleviate symptoms such as joint pain and mood swings associated with menopause.Walnuts, chia seeds, flaxseeds, and fatty fish like salmon, mackerel, and sardines are all great sources of omega-3 fatty acids.

Phytoestrogens are plant-based substances that function in the body similarly to estrogen. Consuming foods rich in phytoestrogens may help alleviate hot flashes, night sweats, and vaginal dryness by modulating hormone levels. Legumes, flaxseeds, sesame seeds, and soy products are good sources of phytoestrogens.

Fiber: Many menopausal women experience digestive issues such as constipation and bloating. Fiber-rich foods can help alleviate these symptoms by promoting regularity and supporting gut health. Whole grains, fruits, vegetables, nuts, and seeds are all excellent sources of dietary fiber.

Antioxidants: Antioxidants help protect cells from damage caused by free radicals and may reduce the risk of chronic diseases associated with aging, such as heart disease and cancer.

Colorful fruits and vegetables, such as berries, citrus fruits, spinach, and bell peppers, are rich in antioxidants and should be included regularly in the diet.

Creating a Balanced Menopause Diet Plan

Now that we understand the key nutrients for menopausal women, let's discuss how to incorporate them into a balanced diet plan:

Emphasize Plant-Based Foods: Aim to fill half your plate with fruits and vegetables at each meal. These foods are rich in vitamins, minerals, fiber, and phytochemicals that support overall health and may help alleviate menopausal symptoms.

Include Lean Protein Sources: Incorporate lean protein sources such as poultry, fish, tofu, legumes, and nuts into your meals to support muscle health and promote satiety.

Choose Healthy Fats: Opt for sources of healthy fats such as avocados, olive oil, nuts, and seeds, which provide essential fatty acids and support heart health.

Limit Processed Foods and Sugars: Minimize your intake of processed foods, sugary snacks, and beverages, as these can exacerbate inflammation and contribute to weight gain and hormonal imbalances.

Keep Yourself Hydrated: To maintain general health and wellbeing and to stay hydrated, sip lots of water throughout the day.

By following these guidelines and incorporating nutrient-rich foods into your diet, you can effectively manage menopausal symptoms and promote optimal health and vitality during this transformative phase of life, and by focusing on nutrient-rich foods and creating a balanced meal plan, you can support your body's

changing needs and alleviate discomfort during
this transitional phase.

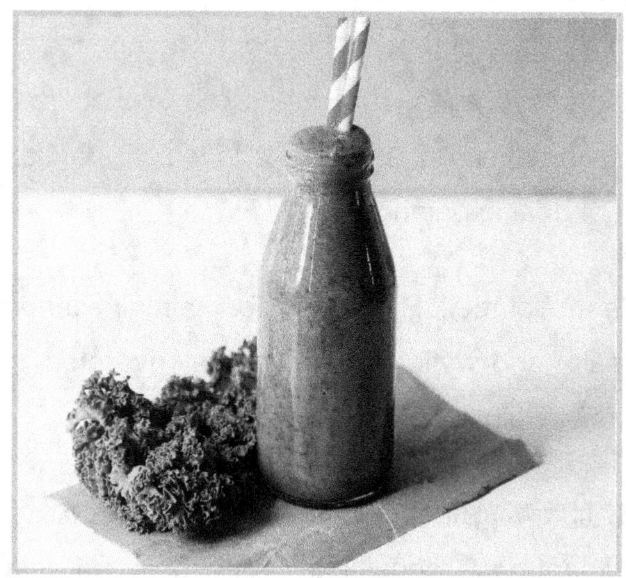

Chapter Three

Essential Nutrients for Menopausal Women

Menopausal women need some essential nutrients to support their health and well-being during this transformative phase of life. From bone health to hormonal balance, these nutrients play crucial roles in alleviating symptoms and promoting vitality as you navigate through menopause.

1. Calcium and Vitamin D:

Calcium and vitamin D are paramount for maintaining strong and healthy bones, especially during menopause when bone density tends to decline. Calcium is the primary mineral responsible for bone structure, while vitamin D helps the body absorb calcium efficiently. Together, they form a formidable duo in preventing osteoporosis and fractures, common concerns for menopausal women.

Good dietary sources of calcium include dairy products like milk, cheese, and yogurt, as well as fortified plant-based alternatives like almond milk and tofu. Leafy greens such as kale, collard greens, and broccoli also contain calcium. However, it's essential to pair calcium-rich foods with vitamin D sources for optimal absorption. Sunlight exposure triggers the body's natural production of vitamin D, but supplements and fortified foods like cereals and orange juice can also provide this vital nutrient.

2. Omega-3 Fatty Acids:

Omega-3 fatty acids are renowned for their anti-inflammatory properties, making them particularly beneficial for managing menopausal symptoms such as joint pain and mood swings. These essential fats also support heart health, cognitive function, and skin integrity, offering a multitude of benefits during menopause and beyond.

Fatty fish like salmon, mackerel, and sardines are rich sources of omega-3s, providing both eicosapentaenoic acid (EPA) and docosahexaenoic acid (DHA). For vegetarians and vegans, flaxseeds, chia seeds, hemp seeds, and walnuts are excellent plant-based alternatives. Incorporating these foods into your diet can help reduce inflammation and promote overall well-being during menopause.

3. Phytoestrogens:

Phytoestrogens are plant compounds that mimic the effects of estrogen in the body, offering relief from menopausal symptoms like hot flashes, night sweats, and vaginal dryness. By binding to estrogen receptors, phytoestrogens can help balance hormone levels and alleviate discomfort during this transitional phase.

Soy products such as tofu, tempeh, and edamame are rich sources of phytoestrogens, particularly a subclass called isoflavones. Other foods like flaxseeds, sesame seeds, lentils, and chickpeas also contain phytoestrogens in varying amounts. Incorporating these plant-based foods into your diet can provide natural relief from menopausal symptoms and support hormonal balance.

4. Fiber:

Fiber is essential for digestive health, promoting regularity, and preventing constipation, a common issue for menopausal women. Additionally, fiber-rich foods help regulate blood sugar levels, support weight management, and reduce the risk of chronic diseases such as heart disease and diabetes.

Whole grains like oats, barley, quinoa, and brown rice are excellent sources of fiber, as are fruits, vegetables, legumes, nuts, and seeds. Aim to include a variety of fiber-rich foods in your diet to support gut health and overall well-being during menopause.

5. Antioxidants:

Antioxidants are compounds that protect cells from oxidative damage caused by free radicals, which can contribute to aging and disease. Menopausal women can benefit from antioxidants' protective effects, reducing the risk of chronic conditions such as heart disease, cancer, and cognitive decline.

Colorful fruits and vegetables are rich sources of antioxidants, including vitamins C and E, beta-carotene, and various phytochemicals. Berries, citrus fruits, spinach, kale, bell peppers, and tomatoes are particularly potent antioxidant powerhouses. Including these nutrient-dense foods in your diet can help support overall health and vitality during menopause.

Here, we have explored the essential nutrients that menopausal women need to support their health and well-being. From calcium and vitamin D for bone health to omega-3 fatty acids for inflammation, these nutrients play critical roles in alleviating symptoms and promoting vitality during this transformative phase of life. By incorporating a variety of nutrient-rich foods into your diet, you can nourish your body and support your journey through menopause with grace and resilience.

Chapter Four

Creating a Balanced Menopause Diet Plan

By incorporating nutrient-rich foods and delicious recipes into your daily meals, you can manage symptoms, maintain energy levels, and promote overall vitality during this transformative phase of life.

Understanding Your Nutritional Needs

Before diving into meal planning, it's essential to understand your unique nutritional needs during menopause. As we discussed in previous chapters, menopausal women require specific nutrients to support bone health, hormonal balance, and overall well-being. These include calcium, vitamin D, omega-3 fatty acids, phytoestrogens, fiber, and antioxidants.

To ensure you're meeting these needs, aim to include a variety of nutrient-rich foods in your diet, focusing on fruits, vegetables, whole grains, lean proteins, and healthy fats. Consider consulting with a registered dietitian or nutritionist to personalize your diet plan based on your age, weight, activity level, and any specific health concerns or dietary restrictions you may have.

Building a Balanced Plate

A balanced diet plan for menopause should consist of a variety of foods from all food groups to ensure you're getting essential nutrients and maintaining overall health. Follow these guidelines to create a balanced plate at each meal:

Fill Half Your Plate with Fruits and Vegetables: Choose a colorful array of fruits and vegetables to provide vitamins, minerals, fiber, and antioxidants. Aim for a mix of leafy greens, cruciferous vegetables, berries, citrus fruits, and other seasonal produce.

Include Lean Proteins: Incorporate lean protein sources such as poultry, fish, tofu, legumes, and nuts to support muscle health and promote satiety. Opt for baked, grilled, or roasted preparations instead of fried or heavily processed options.

Add Whole Grains: Choose whole grains like brown rice, quinoa, oats, barley, and whole wheat bread to provide complex carbohydrates, fiber, and essential nutrients. Avoid refined grains and processed foods, which can spike blood sugar levels and contribute to weight gain.

Don't Forget Healthy Fats: Include sources of healthy fats such as avocados, olive oil, nuts, seeds, and fatty fish to provide essential fatty acids and support heart health.Reduce your intake of processed snacks, fried foods, and fatty meat portions that include saturated and trans fats.

Watch Portion Sizes: Be mindful of portion sizes to prevent overeating and maintain a healthy weight. Use smaller plates, bowls, and utensils to help control portion sizes and avoid mindless eating.

Meal Planning and Preparation

Once you have a basic understanding of your nutritional needs and how to build a balanced plate, it's time to put your meal plan into action. Here are some tips for successful meal planning and preparation:

Make a plan: Set aside some time each week to organize your snacks and meals. Consider your schedule, preferences, and dietary goals when choosing recipes and ingredients.

Batch Cook: Save time and energy by batch cooking staple ingredients like grains, proteins, and vegetables. Cook large batches of quinoa, chicken breast, and roasted vegetables that can be used in multiple meals throughout the week.

Prep Ingredients: Wash, chop, and portion out ingredients in advance to streamline meal preparation. Store prepped ingredients in airtight containers in the refrigerator for easy access when cooking.

Mix and Match: Get creative with your meals by mixing and matching different ingredients and flavors. Use leftovers to create new dishes or repurpose ingredients in salads, stir-fries, soups, and bowls.

Stay Flexible: Be flexible with your meal plan and adjust as needed based on changing circumstances or preferences. Don't be afraid to experiment with new recipes or ingredients to keep things interesting.

Sample Meal Plan

To help you get started, here's a sample meal plan for a day of balanced eating during menopause:

Breakfast: Greek yogurt parfait with mixed berries, almonds, and a drizzle of honey
Mid-Morning Snack: Apple slices with almond butter
Lunch: Quinoa salad with mixed greens, grilled chicken breast, avocado, cherry tomatoes, and balsamic vinaigrette
Afternoon Snack: Carrot sticks with hummus
Dinner: steamed broccoli, roasted sweet potatoes, and baked salmon.
Evening Snack: Dark chocolate squares with a handful of walnuts

By implementing these strategies, you are sure to manage symptoms, maintain energy levels, and promote overall vitality during menopause.

Chapter Five

Quick and Easy Breakfast Recipes for Menopause

We will be exploring a variety of quick and easy breakfast recipes designed to support your health and well-being during menopause in this chapter. Breakfast is often considered the most important meal of the day, providing essential nutrients and energy to kickstart your morning and keep you feeling satisfied until your next meal. With these delicious and nutritious recipes, you'll be able to start your day off right and tackle whatever challenges menopause throws your way.

1. Greek Yogurt Parfait with Mixed Berries and Almonds:

This Greek yogurt parfait is a delicious and satisfying breakfast option that's packed with protein, fiber, and antioxidants. Here's how to make it:

Ingredients:

1/2 cup Greek yogurt

1/4 cup mixed berries (such as strawberries, blueberries, and raspberries)

2 tablespoons sliced almonds

1 teaspoon honey (optional)

Instructions:

In a serving glass or bowl, layer Greek yogurt, mixed berries, and sliced almonds.

If desired, drizzle some honey over the top for a little sweetness.

Serve immediately and enjoy!

2. Avocado Toast with Poached Egg and Spinach:

Avocado toast is a trendy and nutritious breakfast option that's easy to customize with your favorite toppings. Adding a poached egg and spinach boosts the protein and fiber content, making it a satisfying and filling meal. Here's how to make it:

Ingredients:

1 slice whole grain bread, toasted

1/2 ripe avocado, mashed

1 poached egg

Handful of fresh spinach leaves

Salt and pepper to taste

Instructions:

Spread mashed avocado evenly onto the toasted whole grain bread.

Top with fresh spinach leaves.

Carefully place the poached egg on top of the spinach.

Season with salt and pepper to taste.

Serve immediately and enjoy!

3. Overnight Oats with Chia Seeds and Berries:

Overnight oats are a convenient and nutritious breakfast option that can be prepared in advance and enjoyed on busy mornings. The addition of chia seeds provides omega-3 fatty acids and fiber, while the berries add natural sweetness and antioxidants. Here's how to make it:

Ingredients:

1/2 cup rolled oats

1 tablespoon chia seeds

1/2 cup almond milk (or your preferred milk)

1/4 cup mixed berries (such as strawberries, blueberries, and raspberries)

1 tablespoon honey or maple syrup (optional)

Instructions:

In a mason jar or container, combine rolled oats, chia seeds, almond milk, mixed berries, and honey or maple syrup (if using).

Make sure all the ingredients are uniformly distributed by giving the mixture a good stir.

Cover and refrigerate overnight, or for at least 4 hours, to allow the oats and chia seeds to absorb the liquid.

In the morning, give the overnight oats a good stir and add additional milk if desired to achieve your preferred consistency.

Serve cold or warm, and enjoy!

4. Green Smoothie with Spinach, Banana, and Almond Milk:

A green smoothie is a quick and nutritious breakfast option that's perfect for busy mornings. Packed with vitamins, minerals, and fiber, this smoothie will keep you feeling energized and satisfied until your next meal. Here's how to make it:

Ingredients:

1 cup fresh spinach leaves

1 ripe banana

1/2 cup almond milk (or your preferred milk)

1 tablespoon almond butter

1 tablespoon chia seeds

Ice cubes (optional)

Instructions:

In a blender, combine fresh spinach leaves, ripe banana, almond milk, almond butter, and chia seeds.

Blend until smooth and creamy, adding ice cubes if desired to achieve your preferred consistency.

Pour into a glass and enjoy immediately!

5. Veggie Omelette with Tomatoes, Bell Peppers, and Feta Cheese:

An omelette is a versatile and satisfying breakfast option that can be customized with your favorite vegetables and toppings. This veggie omelette is packed with protein, vitamins, and minerals, making it an excellent choice for menopausal women. Here's how to make it:

Ingredients:

2 large eggs

1/4 cup diced tomatoes

1/4 cup diced bell peppers (any color)

2 tablespoons crumbled feta cheese

Salt and pepper to taste

Cooking spray or olive oil

Instructions:

In a small bowl, beat the eggs with a fork until well combined. Season with salt and pepper to taste.

Coat a nonstick skillet with cooking spray or a tiny bit of olive oil and heat it over medium heat.

Pour the beaten eggs into the skillet, swirling to spread evenly.

Cook for 2-3 minutes, or until the eggs begin to set around the edges.

Sprinkle diced tomatoes, bell peppers, and crumbled feta cheese evenly over one half of the omelette.

To create a half-moon shape, delicately fold the remaining omelette over the filling using a spatula.

Cook for an additional 2-3 minutes, or until the eggs are fully cooked and the filling is heated through.

Slide the omelette onto a plate, cut into wedges, and serve immediately.

In this chapter, we've explored a variety of quick and easy breakfast recipes designed to support your health and well-being during menopause. From Greek yogurt parfaits to veggie omelettes, these delicious and nutritious options will keep you feeling satisfied and energized as you navigate through this transformative phase of life. Experiment with different ingredients and flavors to find the breakfast recipes that work best for you, and don't forget to listen to your body's hunger and fullness cues to ensure you're getting the nourishment you need.

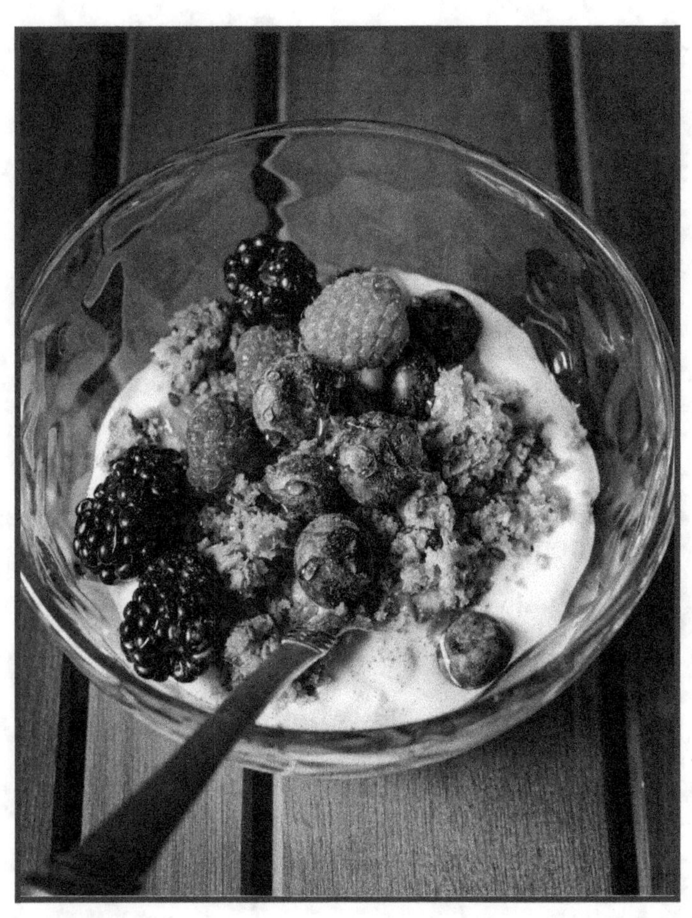

Chapter Six

Nutrient-Rich Lunch Ideas for Menopausal Women

Lunchtime offers an opportunity to refuel your body and replenish your energy levels, especially during menopause when hormonal fluctuations may leave you feeling fatigued or irritable. In this chapter, we'll explore a variety of nutrient-rich lunch ideas designed to nourish your body and support your well-being during this transformative phase of life.

1. Quinoa Salad with Grilled Chicken and Avocado:

Quinoa is a versatile and nutrient-rich grain that serves as the perfect base for a satisfying lunch salad. Packed with protein, fiber, and essential vitamins and minerals, quinoa provides long-lasting energy to keep you feeling full and satisfied throughout the afternoon. Pair it with grilled chicken for lean protein and avocado for healthy fats, and you've got a delicious and balanced meal that's perfect for menopausal women.

To make this quinoa salad, start by cooking quinoa according to package instructions and letting it cool. Meanwhile, season chicken breasts with your favorite herbs and spices and grill until cooked through. Once the quinoa and chicken are ready, simply toss them together with diced avocado, cherry tomatoes, cucumber, and fresh herbs like cilantro or parsley. Drizzle with a simple vinaigrette made from olive oil, lemon juice, and Dijon mustard, and enjoy a hearty and nutritious lunch that's as satisfying as it is delicious.

2. Lentil Soup with Spinach and Turmeric:

Lentil soup is a comforting and nourishing option for lunch, especially during the colder months or when you're craving something warm and satisfying. Lentils are an excellent source of plant-based protein, fiber, and iron, making them a great choice for menopausal women who may be at risk of iron deficiency due to hormonal changes. Adding spinach to the soup provides additional vitamins and minerals, while turmeric adds anti-inflammatory properties and a warm, earthy flavor.

To make this lentil soup, start by sautéing diced onions, carrots, and celery in olive oil until softened. Add minced garlic, ground turmeric, cumin, and coriander, and cook until fragrant. Then, add dried lentils, vegetable broth, and diced tomatoes, and simmer until the lentils are tender. Stir in chopped spinach and cook until wilted, then season with salt and pepper to taste. Serve the soup hot with a slice of whole grain bread or a side salad for a complete and satisfying meal.

3. Salmon Salad with Quinoa and Citrus Dressing:

Salmon is rich in omega-3 fatty acids, which have been shown to reduce inflammation and support a healthy heart, making it an excellent choice for menopausal women. Pairing it with quinoa, a nutrient-rich grain, and a citrusy dressing adds flavor and freshness to this satisfying lunch salad.

To make this salmon salad, start by seasoning salmon fillets with salt, pepper, and a squeeze of lemon juice, then bake or grill until cooked through. As you wait, prepare the quinoa per the directions on the package and allow it to cool. Once the salmon and quinoa are ready, simply toss them together with mixed greens, sliced avocado, cherry tomatoes, and thinly sliced red onion. For the dressing, whisk together olive oil, fresh lemon juice, Dijon mustard, honey, and minced garlic until emulsified. Drizzle the dressing over the salad and toss to coat evenly, then serve immediately for a delicious and nutritious lunch that's bursting with flavor.

4. Brown rice and vegetable stir-fry with tofu:

Stir-fries are a quick and easy lunch option that's perfect for busy days or when you're short on time. Packed with colorful vegetables, protein-rich tofu, and hearty brown rice, this veggie stir-fry provides a satisfying and nutritious meal that's sure to keep you feeling full and energized.

To make this veggie stir-fry, start by pressing tofu to remove excess moisture, then dice it into cubes. Sauté tofu in a skillet with olive oil until golden brown and crispy on all sides, then set aside. In the same skillet, stir-fry your favorite vegetables, such as bell peppers, broccoli, snap peas, carrots, and mushrooms, until tender-crisp. Add minced garlic, ginger, and soy sauce for flavor, then toss in the cooked tofu and cooked brown rice until heated through. Serve the stir-fry hot with a sprinkle of sesame seeds or chopped green onions for extra flavor and enjoy a delicious and nutritious lunch that's packed with plant-based goodness.

5. Chickpea Salad with Roasted Vegetables and Tahini Dressing:

Chickpeas are a versatile and nutrient-rich legume that serves as the perfect base for a satisfying lunch salad. Packed with protein, fiber, and essential vitamins and minerals, chickpeas provide long-lasting energy to keep you feeling full and satisfied throughout the afternoon. Pair them with roasted vegetables for added flavor and texture, and drizzle with a creamy tahini dressing for a delicious and nutritious meal that's perfect for menopausal women.

To make this chickpea salad, start by roasting your favorite vegetables, such as cherry tomatoes, bell peppers, zucchini, and red onion, until caramelized and tender.

Meanwhile, rinse and drain canned chickpeas and toss them with olive oil, salt, pepper, and your favorite herbs and spices.Bake the chickpeas in the oven until they become golden brown and crispy. Once the vegetables and chickpeas are ready, simply toss them together with mixed greens, sliced cucumber, and fresh herbs like parsley or cilantro. For the dressing, whisk together tahini, lemon juice, garlic, and water until smooth and creamy, then drizzle over the salad and toss to coat evenly. Serve the salad immediately for a delicious and nutritious lunch that's as satisfying as it is flavorful.

We've explored a variety of nutrient-rich lunch ideas designed to support your health and well-being during menopause. From quinoa salad with grilled chicken to lentil soup with spinach and turmeric, these delicious and nutritious recipes will keep you feeling satisfied and energized as you navigate through this transformative phase of life. Experiment with different ingredients and flavors to find the lunch recipes that work best for you, and don't forget to listen to your body's hunger and fullness cues to ensure you're getting the nourishment you need.

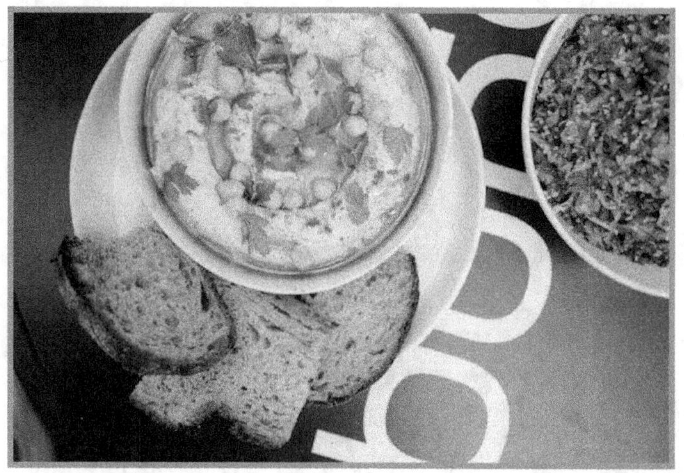

Chapter Seven

Delicious Dinners to Support Hormonal Balance

Dinner time is an opportunity to unwind and nourish your body after a long day, especially during menopause when hormonal changes may affect your appetite and energy levels. In this chapter, we'll explore a variety of hearty dinner recipes designed to provide comfort, satisfaction, and essential nutrients for menopausal women. From comforting soups to satisfying one-pan meals, these recipes are sure to become staples in your meal rotation.

1. Butternut Squash Soup with Turmeric and Ginger:

Butternut squash soup is a comforting and nutritious option for dinner, particularly during the colder months or when you're craving something warm and satisfying. Butternut squash is rich in vitamins, minerals, and antioxidants, while turmeric and ginger add anti-inflammatory properties and a warm, earthy flavor. Here's how to make it:

Ingredients:

One medium-sized butternut squash, chopped, seeded, and skinned

1 onion, diced

2 cloves garlic, minced

1-inch piece of fresh ginger, grated

1 teaspoon ground turmeric

4 cups vegetable broth

1 can (14 oz) coconut milk

Salt and pepper to taste

Fresh cilantro for garnish (optional)

Instructions:

In a large pot, sauté diced onion in olive oil until softened.

Add minced garlic, grated ginger, and ground turmeric, and cook until fragrant.

Add diced butternut squash and vegetable broth to the pot, and bring to a simmer.

Cook until the squash is tender, about 20-25 minutes.

Blend the soup with an immersion blender until it's creamy and smooth.

Add the coconut milk and taste-test to adjust the seasoning.

If preferred, top the heated dish with freshly chopped cilantro.

2. Baked Salmon with Roasted Vegetables:

Salmon is an excellent source of omega-3 fatty acids, which have been shown to reduce inflammation and support a healthy heart, making it an ideal choice for menopausal women. Pairing it with roasted vegetables creates a balanced and satisfying meal that's perfect for busy weeknights. Here's how to make it:

Ingredients:

4 salmon fillets

1 pound mixed vegetables (such as carrots, broccoli, and bell peppers), chopped

2 tablespoons olive oil

2 cloves garlic, minced

1 teaspoon dried thyme

Salt and pepper to taste

Lemon wedges for serving

Instructions:

Preheat the oven to 400°F (200°C).

Arrange the salmon fillets on a parchment paper-lined baking pan.

In a large bowl, toss chopped vegetables with olive oil, minced garlic, dried thyme, salt, and pepper.

Spread vegetables evenly around the salmon fillets on the baking sheet.

Bake in the preheated oven for 15-20 minutes, or until salmon is cooked through and vegetables are tender.

Present the salmon hot, along with lemon wedges for squeezing.

3. One-Pot Chicken and Vegetable Curry:

Curry is a flavorful and comforting dish that's perfect for warming up on chilly evenings. This one-pot chicken and vegetable curry is packed with protein, fiber, and essential nutrients, making it an excellent choice for menopausal women. Here's how to make it:

Ingredients:

1 tablespoon coconut oil

1 onion, diced

2 cloves garlic, minced

1-inch piece of fresh ginger, grated

2 tablespoons curry powder

1 can (14 oz) diced tomatoes

1 can (14 oz) coconut milk

2 cups diced cooked chicken breast

2 cups mixed vegetables (such as carrots, peas, and bell peppers)

Salt and pepper to taste

Fresh cilantro for garnish (optional)

Cooked rice or naan bread for serving

Instructions:

In a large pot or skillet, heat coconut oil over medium heat.

Add diced onion, minced garlic, and grated ginger, and cook until softened.

Stir in curry powder and cook until fragrant.

Add diced tomatoes and coconut milk to the pot, and bring to a simmer.

Add diced cooked chicken breast and mixed vegetables to the pot, and simmer until heated through.

Season with salt and pepper to taste.

Serve hot, garnished with fresh cilantro if desired, and with cooked rice or naan bread on the side.

4. Lentil and Vegetable Stir-Fry:

Stir-fries are a quick and easy dinner option that's perfect for busy weeknights. This lentil and vegetable stir-fry is packed with plant-based protein, fiber, and essential nutrients, making it a satisfying and nutritious meal for menopausal women. Here's how to make it:

Ingredients:

1 cup dried lentils, rinsed and drained

2 cups vegetable broth

2 tablespoons olive oil

1 onion, sliced

2 cloves garlic, minced

Two cups of sliced mixed veggies, including bell peppers, broccoli, and snap peas

2 tablespoons soy sauce

1 tablespoon rice vinegar

1 teaspoon sesame oil

Cooked brown rice for serving

Instructions:

In a medium saucepan, combine dried lentils and vegetable broth, and bring to a boil.

Reduce heat to low, cover, and simmer until lentils are tender, about 20-25 minutes.

Meanwhile, heat olive oil in a large skillet or wok over medium-high heat.

Add sliced onion and minced garlic to the skillet, and cook until softened.

Add mixed vegetables to the skillet, and stir-fry until tender-crisp.

Stir in cooked lentils, soy sauce, rice vinegar, and sesame oil, and cook until heated through.

Serve hot, with cooked brown rice on the side.

5. Quinoa Stuffed Bell Peppers:

Stuffed bell peppers are a delicious and nutritious dinner option that's perfect for menopausal women. This recipe features quinoa, a protein-rich grain, combined with vegetables, herbs, and spices, all stuffed inside colorful bell peppers and baked to perfection. Here's how to make it:

Ingredients:

4 bell peppers, halved and seeds removed

1 cup cooked quinoa

One can (14.2 oz) of rinsed and drained black beans

1 cup corn kernels (fresh or frozen)

1 cup diced tomatoes

1/2 cup diced onion

2 cloves garlic, minced

1 teaspoon ground cumin

1 teaspoon chili powder

Salt and pepper to taste

Shredded cheese for topping (optional)

Fresh cilantro for garnish (optional)

Instructions:

Preheat the oven to 375°F (190°C).

Place bell pepper halves cut side up in a baking dish.

In a large bowl, combine cooked quinoa, black beans, corn kernels, diced tomatoes, diced onion, minced garlic, ground cumin, chili powder, salt, and pepper.

Spoon quinoa mixture evenly into each bell pepper half.

Cover the baking dish with aluminum foil and bake in the preheated oven for 25-30 minutes, or until peppers are tender.

Remove foil, sprinkle stuffed peppers with shredded cheese if desired, and return to the oven for an additional 5 minutes, or until the cheese is melted and bubbly.

If preferred, top the heated dish with freshly chopped cilantro.

Having explored a variety of hearty dinner recipes designed to provide comfort, satisfaction, and essential nutrients for menopausal women, from comforting soups to satisfying one-pan meals, these recipes are sure to become staples in your meal rotation. Experiment with different ingredients and flavors to find the dinner recipes that work best for you, and don't forget to listen to your body's hunger and fullness cues to ensure you're getting the nourishment you need.

Chapter Eight

Snacks and Treats for Menopausal Cravings

Snacking can be an important part of a balanced diet, providing energy and essential nutrients between meals. However, finding nutritious and satisfying snacks can be challenging, especially during menopause when hormonal changes may affect appetite and cravings. Here we'll explore a variety of snack ideas specifically tailored to support menopausal health. From protein-rich options to fiber-packed treats, these snacks will help you stay energized, satisfied, and nourished throughout the day.

1. Greek Yogurt with Berries and Almonds:

Greek yogurt is a nutrient-rich snack that's packed with protein, calcium, and probiotics, making it an excellent choice for menopausal women. Pairing it with fresh berries adds natural sweetness, fiber, and antioxidants, while almonds provide healthy fats and crunch. Here's how to make it:

Ingredients:

1/2 cup Greek yogurt

1/4 cup mixed berries (such as strawberries, blueberries, and raspberries)

2 tablespoons sliced almonds

Instructions:

In a small bowl, spoon Greek yogurt.

Top with mixed berries and sliced almonds.

Enjoy immediately as a satisfying and nutritious snack.

2. Hummus with Carrot Sticks and Whole Grain Crackers:

Hummus is a creamy and flavorful dip made from chickpeas, tahini, olive oil, lemon juice, and garlic, making it a nutritious and satisfying snack option for menopausal women. Pairing it with carrot sticks and whole grain crackers adds crunch, fiber, and additional nutrients. Here's how to make it:

Ingredients:

1/4 cup hummus

1 medium carrot, cut into sticks

Whole grain crackers

Instructions:

Spoon hummus into a small bowl.

Arrange carrot sticks and whole grain crackers on a plate.

Dip carrot sticks and crackers into hummus and enjoy as a delicious and nutritious snack.

3. Cottage Cheese with Pineapple and Walnuts:

Cottage cheese is a protein-rich snack that's low in calories and high in calcium, making it an excellent choice for menopausal women. Pairing it with fresh pineapple adds natural sweetness and vitamin C, while walnuts provide healthy fats and crunch. Here's how to make it:

Ingredients:

1/2 cup cottage cheese

1/2 cup fresh pineapple chunks

2 tablespoons chopped walnuts

Instructions:

Spoon cottage cheese into a small bowl.

Top with fresh pineapple chunks and chopped walnuts.

Enjoy immediately as a satisfying and nutritious snack.

4. Avocado Toast with Cherry Tomatoes and Hemp Seeds:

Avocado toast is a trendy and nutritious snack option that's easy to customize with your favorite toppings. Avocado provides healthy fats and fiber, while cherry tomatoes add sweetness and hemp seeds contribute protein and omega-3 fatty acids. Here's how to make it:

Ingredients:

1 slice whole grain bread, toasted

1/2 ripe avocado, mashed

4-5 cherry tomatoes, sliced

1 tablespoon hemp seeds

Instructions:

Spread mashed avocado evenly onto the toasted whole grain bread.

Top the avocado with a layer of sliced cherry tomatoes.

Sprinkle hemp seeds over the cherry tomatoes.

Savor it right away as a tasty and wholesome snack.

5. Nuts & Dried Fruit Trail Mix:

Trail mix is a convenient and portable snack option that's perfect for on-the-go menopausal women. Combining dried fruit and nuts provides a satisfying mix of sweetness, crunch, protein, and healthy fats. Here's how to make it:

Ingredients:

1/4 cup dried cranberries

1/4 cup dried apricots, chopped

1/4 cup almonds

1/4 cup cashews

1/4 cup pumpkin seeds

Instructions:

In a small bowl, combine dried cranberries, chopped dried apricots, almonds, cashews, and pumpkin seeds.

Mix well to combine.

Portion trail mix into small resealable bags for a convenient and portable snack.

6. Veggie Sticks with Hummus Dip:

Veggie sticks with hummus dip are a nutritious and satisfying snack option that's perfect for menopausal women. Crunchy vegetables like carrots, cucumber, celery, and bell peppers provide fiber, vitamins, and minerals, while hummus adds protein and flavor. Here's how to make it:

Ingredients:

Assorted veggie sticks (carrots, cucumber, celery, bell peppers)

1/4 cup hummus

Instructions:

Wash and cut assorted vegetables into sticks.

Spoon hummus into a small bowl.

Dip veggie sticks into hummus and enjoy as a nutritious and satisfying snack.

7. Edamame with Sea Salt:

Edamame is a protein-rich snack that's packed with fiber, vitamins, and minerals, making it an excellent choice for menopausal women. Sprinkling it with sea salt adds flavor and enhances its natural sweetness. Here's how to make it:

Ingredients:

1 cup cooked edamame

Sea salt to taste

Instructions:

Cook edamame according to package instructions.

Drain and rinse edamame under cold water.

Sprinkle edamame with sea salt to taste.

Enjoy immediately as a nutritious and satisfying snack.

8. Apple Slices with Almond Butter:

Apple slices with almond butter are a simple and delicious snack option that's perfect for menopausal women. Apples provide fiber, vitamins, and antioxidants, while almond butter adds protein, healthy fats, and flavor. Here's how to make it:

Ingredients:

1 medium apple, sliced

2 tablespoons almond butter

Instructions:

Wash and core the apple, then slice into wedges.

Spread almond butter onto apple slices.

Enjoy immediately as a satisfying and nutritious snack.

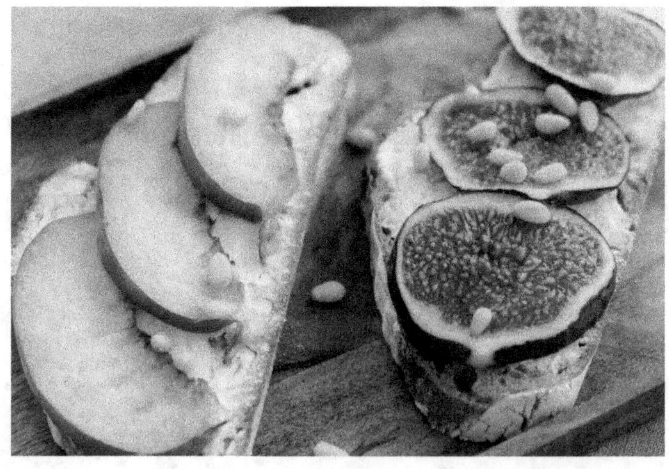

Chapter Nine

Beverages to Stay Hydrated and Healthy During Menopause

Hydration is essential for overall health and well-being, especially during menopause. As hormonal changes occur, women may experience symptoms such as hot flashes, night sweats, and mood swings, which can affect hydration levels and fluid balance in the body. Here, we'll explore a variety of beverages and hydration strategies specifically tailored to help menopausal women stay hydrated and healthy during this transformative phase of life.

Understanding Hydration Needs During Menopause

Before diving into specific beverages and hydration strategies, it's important to understand the unique hydration needs of menopausal women. Hormonal changes during menopause can lead to an increased risk of dehydration due to symptoms like hot flashes and night sweats, which can cause excessive sweating and fluid loss. Additionally, aging itself can affect the body's ability to retain water and regulate thirst.

During menopause, the body's hydration needs may increase, making it crucial to prioritize fluid intake throughout the day. Dehydration can exacerbate symptoms such as fatigue, headaches, and dry skin, so staying adequately hydrated is essential for overall health and well-being.

Key Hydration Strategies

Drink Water Regularly: Water is the best way to stay hydrated, so aim to drink plenty of fluids throughout the day. Keep a water bottle with you wherever you go, and take sips regularly to stay hydrated.

Monitor Urine Color: One way to gauge hydration levels is by monitoring the color of your urine. Pale or light yellow urine indicates adequate hydration, while dark yellow or amber-colored urine may signal dehydration.

Pay Attention to Thirst Signals: As we age, our sense of thirst may become less sensitive. Therefore, it's important to pay attention to thirst signals and drink water even if you don't feel thirsty.

Eat Hydrating Foods: In addition to beverages, certain foods can contribute to hydration. Fruits and vegetables with high water content, such as watermelon, cucumber, oranges, and strawberries, can help boost hydration levels.

Limit Dehydrating Beverages: Some beverages, such as caffeinated drinks and alcohol, can have diuretic effects and increase fluid loss. While it's okay to enjoy these beverages in moderation, be mindful of their potential impact on hydration levels.

Now, let's explore some specific beverages that can help menopausal women stay hydrated and healthy:

1. Infused Water:

Infused water is a refreshing and flavorful way to stay hydrated without added sugars or calories. Simply add sliced fruits, vegetables, or herbs to a pitcher of water and let it infuse for a few hours in the refrigerator. Some delicious combinations to try include cucumber and mint, lemon and ginger, or strawberry and basil. Infused water not only provides hydration but also adds vitamins, minerals, and antioxidants to your diet.

2. Herbal Teas:

Herbal teas are caffeine-free and hydrating, making them an excellent choice for menopausal women. Herbal teas come in a variety of flavors and can provide soothing benefits for symptoms like hot flashes and anxiety. Chamomile tea is known for its calming properties, while peppermint tea can aid digestion and relieve bloating. Experiment with different herbal teas to find flavors that you enjoy and incorporate them into your daily hydration routine.

3. Coconut Water:

Coconut water is a natural source of electrolytes, including potassium, magnesium, and sodium, making it an excellent choice for replenishing fluids and electrolytes lost through sweating. Unlike sugary sports drinks, coconut water is low in calories and contains no added sugars, making it a healthier option for hydration. Enjoy coconut water on its own or use it as a base for smoothies and hydration drinks.

4. Green Smoothies:

Green smoothies are a nutrient-rich way to stay hydrated while boosting your intake of fruits and vegetables. Blend leafy greens like spinach or kale with hydrating fruits like cucumber, celery, and pineapple, along with a splash of water or coconut water. You can also add protein-rich ingredients like Greek yogurt or protein powder for added staying power. Green smoothies are not only hydrating but also provide essential vitamins, minerals, and antioxidants to support overall health during menopause.

5. Electrolyte Drinks:

Electrolyte drinks can help replenish fluids and essential minerals lost through sweating, making them beneficial for menopausal women experiencing symptoms like hot flashes and night sweats. Look for electrolyte drinks that are low in sugar and contain a balanced blend of electrolytes like potassium, magnesium, and sodium. You can also make your own electrolyte drink at home by mixing coconut water with a pinch of sea salt and a squeeze of lemon or lime juice.

Staying hydrated is essential for overall health and well-being, especially during menopause when hormonal changes can affect fluid balance in the body. By prioritizing hydration and incorporating a variety of hydrating beverages into your daily routine, you can support your health and manage symptoms more effectively. Experiment with different beverages, monitor your fluid intake, and listen to your body's thirst signals to ensure you're staying adequately hydrated throughout the day. With these hydration strategies, you can stay hydrated and healthy during menopause, allowing you to embrace this transformative phase of life with vitality and well-being.

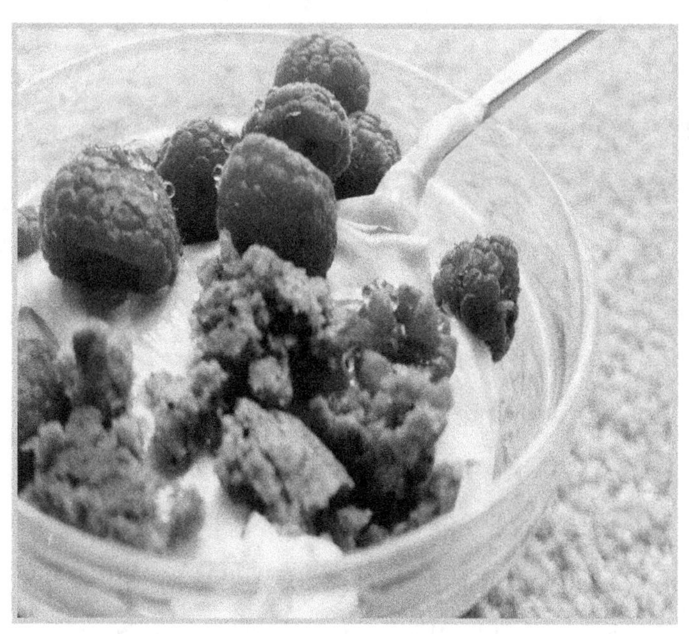

Chapter Ten

Meal Prep Tips for Simplifying Your Menopause Diet Journey

Meal prep is a valuable tool for simplifying your menopause diet journey. As hormonal changes occur during menopause, maintaining a healthy and balanced diet becomes increasingly important for managing symptoms and supporting overall well-being. However, busy schedules and fluctuating energy levels can make it challenging to prepare nutritious meals consistently. In this chapter, we'll explore a variety of meal prep tips and strategies to help you streamline your menopause diet journey, saving time and effort while nourishing your body with delicious and wholesome foods.

Understanding the Importance of Meal Prep During Menopause

Before diving into meal prep tips, it's essential to understand why meal prep is particularly beneficial during menopause. Hormonal changes during menopause can impact appetite, metabolism, and energy levels, making it essential to prioritize nutrition and meal planning. By preparing meals and snacks in advance, you can ensure that you have healthy options readily available, reducing the temptation to reach for convenience foods that may be high in sugar, salt, or unhealthy fats.

Meal prep also allows you to control portion sizes and ingredients, making it easier to stick to your dietary goals and manage weight fluctuations that may occur during menopause. Additionally, having pre-prepared meals on hand can alleviate stress and decision fatigue, allowing you to focus on other aspects of your health and well-being during this transitional phase of life.

Key Meal Prep Tips for Menopausal Women

Plan Your Meals Weekly: Take some time at the beginning of each week to plan your meals for the upcoming days. Consider your schedule, dietary preferences, and nutritional needs when selecting recipes. Planning your meals in advance can help you create a shopping list and ensure that you have all the ingredients you need on hand.

Batch Cooking: Batch cooking involves preparing large quantities of food at once and portioning it out for future meals. Choose one or two days a week to dedicate to batch cooking, and prepare staples like grains, proteins, and vegetables in bulk. Store individual portions in containers or freezer bags for easy grab-and-go meals throughout the week.

Focus on Versatile Ingredients: Choose versatile ingredients that can be used in multiple recipes to save time and reduce waste. For example, roasted vegetables can be added to salads, grain bowls, or wraps, while cooked quinoa or brown rice can serve as a base for various dishes. By incorporating versatile ingredients into your meal prep, you can create a variety of meals without the need for extensive cooking each day.

Use Time-Saving Kitchen Tools: Invest in time-saving kitchen tools and appliances to streamline your meal prep process. Tools like a slow cooker, Instant Pot, or food processor can help you prepare meals more efficiently, allowing you to spend less time in the kitchen. Additionally, consider pre-cutting vegetables, pre-cooking grains, or using frozen fruits and vegetables to save time on meal prep.

Pre-Portion Snacks: Take the time to pre-portion snacks like nuts, seeds, fruits, and yogurt into individual servings. Having pre-portioned snacks readily available makes it easier to make healthier choices throughout the day and prevents overeating. Store pre-portioned snacks in grab-and-go containers or snack bags for convenience.

Create a Meal Prep Schedule: Establish a meal prep schedule that works for your lifestyle and preferences. Whether you prefer to meal prep on weekends or dedicate a few hours each evening to cooking, consistency is key. Set aside designated time for meal prep each week and stick to your schedule to ensure that you have nutritious meals and snacks available when you need them.

Experiment with Make-Ahead Freezer Meals: Consider incorporating make-ahead freezer meals into your meal prep routine. Prepare large batches of soups, stews, casseroles, or lasagnas and freeze them in individual portions for future use. Freezer meals can be a lifesaver on busy days when you don't have time to cook, providing a convenient and nutritious option for meals at a moment's notice.

Don't Forget About Breakfast: Breakfast is an important meal, especially during menopause when stable energy levels are essential for managing symptoms. Prepare make-ahead breakfast options like overnight oats, breakfast burritos, or egg muffins that can be quickly reheated or enjoyed cold in the morning. Having breakfast ready to go can set the tone for a healthy and energized day ahead.

By planning your meals weekly, batch cooking, focusing on versatile ingredients, and using time-saving kitchen tools, you can streamline your meal prep process and ensure that you have nutritious meals and snacks readily available throughout the week. Experiment with different meal prep techniques to find what works best for you and your lifestyle. With a little planning and preparation, you can nourish your body with delicious and wholesome foods, supporting your health and well-being during this transformative phase of life. Embrace the power of meal prep and enjoy the benefits of simplified and stress-free eating during menopause.

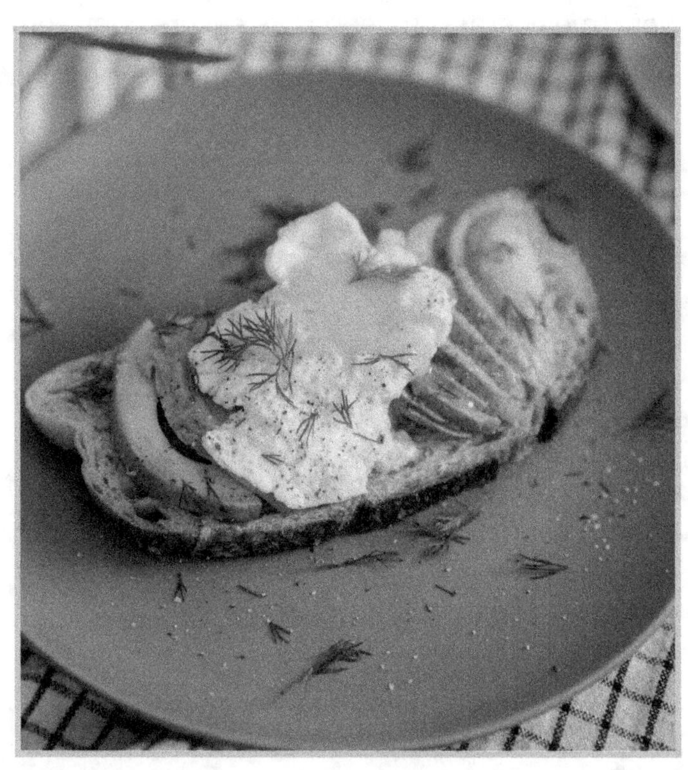

Conclusion

Well done for starting down the path to a better, healthier version of yourself. By incorporating these menopause diet recipes into your daily life, you're not only nourishing your body, but also empowering yourself to take control of your health during this significant life transition.

Remember, menopause is a natural part of life, and with the right tools and mindset, you can thrive during this phase. The recipes in this book are designed to support your physical and emotional well-being, helping to alleviate symptoms and improve your overall quality of life.

As you continue on this journey, remember to be kind to yourself, listen to your body, and celebrate your strength and resilience. Don't be afraid to seek support from loved ones, healthcare professionals, or online communities – you are not alone!

By embracing these recipes and the principles of healthy eating, you're investing in your long-term health and happiness. You got this! You are capable of navigating menopause with grace, confidence, and a full plate of delicious, nourishing food.

Wishing you a vibrant, healthy, and joyful journey ahead!

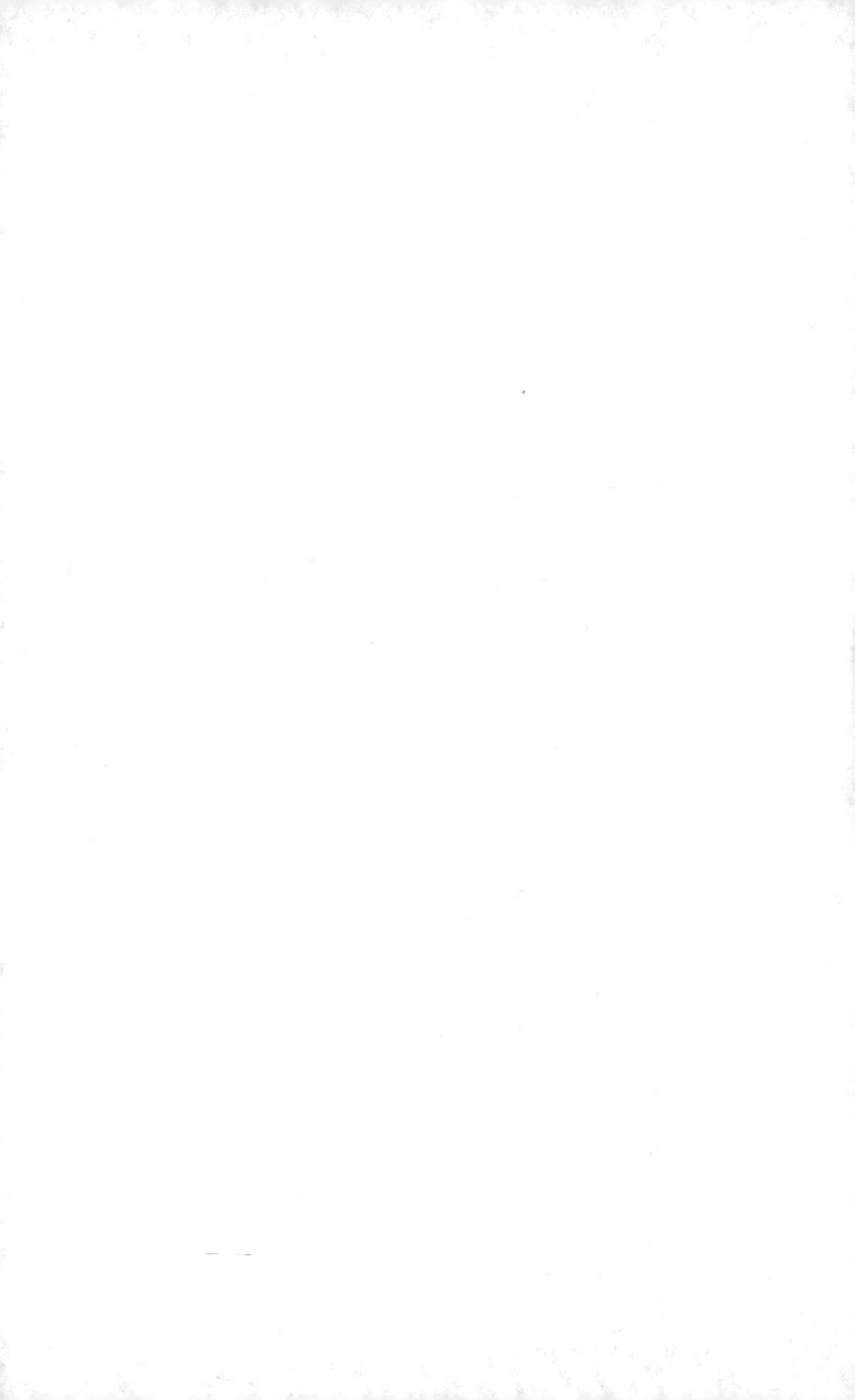

www.ingramcontent.com/pod-product-compliance
Lightning Source LLC
Chambersburg PA
CBHW051831250726
48659CB00005B/1784